CHOOSING THE RIGHT DIET FOR SUCCESS

(WITH LASTING RESULTS)

By

Pennie Mae Cartawick

Important Legal Disclaimer

The information presented in this book reflects the author's opinions and is by no way intended as medical advice or as a substitute for medical counseling. This information should be used in conjunction with the guidance and care of your physician. Consult your physician before beginning any exercise and nutrition program.

The author has made every effort to supply accurate information in the creation of this book. The author offers no warranty and accepts no responsibility for any loss or damages of any kind that may be incurred by the reader as a result of actions arising from the use of the contents in this book. If you choose not to obtain the consent of your physician and/or work with your physician throughout the duration of your time using the recommendations in this book, you are agreeing to accept full responsibility for your actions.

Table of Contents

Introduction

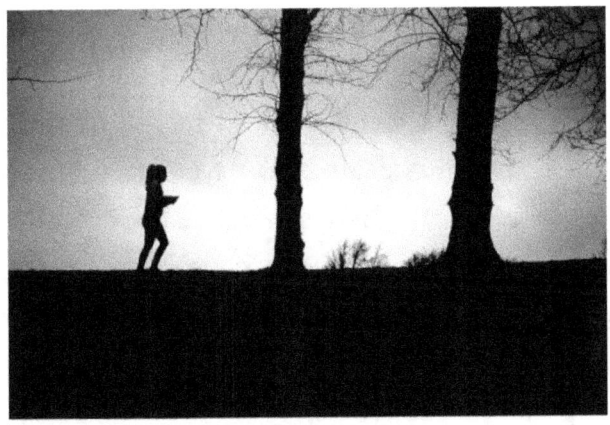

Whether you are thinking of going on a diet for the first time, have been on diets in the past that you couldn't stick to or worked really hard to achieve your goal only to gain the weight back again, it can be frustrating, and your confidence of trying again keeps going away. This book is intended to help choose the right diet for your own personal success and to help you achieve your goal and, more importantly, keep those pesky pounds away for good. Dieting doesn't have to be a chore; it can be part of a wonderful lifestyle with lasting results. This introduction has a few examples of supplements and exercise programs to think about. The book contents contain insight into other various methods for choosing the right diet and fitness strategies that will work best for you so losing weight and maintaining it can be an enjoyable, lifelong experience.

Weight loss is the one of the oldest health and fitness mantras in the modern world and every man and woman yearns to have an up-to-the-minute look that will draw all the attention to him or her. It is everyone's desire to look sexier, healthier and more fit. However, nothing comes to us on a silver plate. If you visualize losing some pounds, then this book can help to achieve your goal and give insight into choosing an effective weight loss and exercise program. Broadly speaking, weight loss procedures can involve exercises or can be exercise free. Here are a few examples of both of them.

Weight loss supplements

There is no denying that dietary supplements are the cornerstone of natural, exercise-free weight loss procedures. They work by burning fat and reducing the body's BMR (Basal Metabolic Rate). It is also worth noting that most weight loss supplements in their pure forms are safe, and the side effects associated with some of them can be attributed to impurities or failure to follow the doctor's advice.

HCG diet protocols

The HCG diet protocol is a natural, exercise-free weight loss method based on high Human Chorionic Gonadotropin (HCG) hormone and a 500-calorie diet. HCG protocols normally come in four phases that run for 23-40 days, after which the process can be repeated. A person can decide to use either an injection or sublingual HCG option and exercising is not required, though mild exercises will do no harm.

Though HCG protocols are generally safe, most users have complained of headache, irritability, painful injections, diarrhea, constipation and nausea. Most likely, these side effects are brought about by using scam products. Additionally, most users, especially those suffering from gall bladder ailments, do not relish the idea of dietary restrictions.

Garcinia Cambogia

The effectiveness of this supplement stems from one of its ingredients, Hydroxycitric Acid (HCA), which is very effective in reducing appetite and lowering cholesterol levels, as well as increasing fat metabolism.

Garcinia Cambogia can be in the form of powder or pills. It is generally a safe supplement in its pure form but its side effects can be attributed to over-dosage, under-dosage or failure to follow the physician's prescriptions. Some of these side effects include nausea, headache, digestive tract discomfort, as well as some laxative effects.

Green coffee bean extract

Green coffee bean extract is beneficial in reducing both blood pressure and weight. This is because the beans are unroasted, and they contain high levels of chlorogenic acid (an antioxidant), which inhibits the release of glucose from the liver to the bloodstream, thereby reducing the body's weight. This acid also impacts positively on blood sugar and metabolism in human beings.

Several scholars, health practitioners and researchers have spent sleepless nights trying to unearth the tidbits of physical, clinical or medicinal side effects of the green coffee bean extract, to no avail.

This is not all. Other weight loss supplements include Beta-Glucan CLA (Conjugated Linoleic Acid), Chitosan, whey protein, mango seed fiber, white bean extract, chia, resveratrol, capsaicin, hoodia, and apple cider vinegar. Each of these supplements has its unique pros.

Slimming creams and lotions may also be used to sculpt some parts of the body. For instance, women give their legs a slim and sexy look using the recently released Once All Ginger Leg Slimming Cream Fat Reducing Body Cream (released in October 2013). As per the status quo, this cream does not have side effects.

As observed above, weight loss supplements do not come without side effects. These effects may be mild or far-reaching and catastrophic, and therefore they need to be avoided at all costs. This leads us to the second weight loss method: exercise.

Exercise and weight loss

Exercise may be tiring but it will definitely satisfy your beauty needs. Just try these exercises and look at yourself into the mirror. You will be a new creation: gorgeous and confident.

Pilates

Pilates can be described as a physical fitness program encompassing six principles: concentration, control, core or center, smooth flow, precision and breathing. Designed and implemented by Joseph Pilate, this corrective program is based on the control of the body's fitness, hence the original term "controllogy."

There are several advantages of Pilates. First, it leads to physical and mental body conditioning and awareness. The core or center principle ensures development of a strong center or focal point and strong, balanced musculature. Pilates aligns the spinal cord and pelvic girdle and improves the breathing system.

Yoga

Yoga is based on five principles, namely: proper exercise, correct breathing, proper diet, positive thinking and complete relaxation.

Yoga and Pilates overlap in several situations. For instance, they are both transformational and their outcomes are more or less similar. They both lead to body-mind awareness and connection, but yoga also encompasses a spiritual connection. These similarities notwithstanding, there are unique factors of each method. The most obvious difference is that yoga is a "practice" while Pilates is a "workout," but it is arguable that frequent workout practice makes perfect (pardon the irony and pun). Both of these exercises also have different origins. Pilates was designed by Joseph Pilates while yoga is based on ancient Indian culture.

Cross Fit

Cross Fit is a multi-dimensional fitness training methodology developed by Greg Glassman which focuses on speed, strength and gymnastics. It is fit, efficient and safe for both men and women. It improves general body fitness, movement and dietary practices. Being a rigorous and intense workout, it ensures that no body part is left untrained, leading to enhanced sport performance. To add color to the already good package, this training is cheap and it can be done at home, allowing the participant to work at the convenience of his/her own supervision. Cross Fit also leads to cardiorespiratory fitness, stamina, flexibility, agility, balance, accuracy, coordination, endurance and longevity.

Pilates, yoga and Cross Fit are planned exercises. Other unplanned exercises include swimming, walking, biking, skiing, cross country and any household chores. These exercises are also influential in weight loss programs.

Both exercise and exercise-free weight loss programs depend on a set of guidelines for them to work and to avoid a "square peg in a round hole" situation. First, a weight loss participant must choose the weight loss procedure that works for them. If supplements work for you, then follow your physician's advice and recommendation religiously. Do not violate the dosage instructions and prescriptions, and ensure that there are no filler or additive ingredients in the supplements.

On the other hand, if exercise works for you, then keep in mind that any weight loss exercise program is elaborate and it requires total commitment until you attain the so-called noticeable difference threshold. Moreover, your body constantly rejects the change that you desire and this should not pour cold water on your efforts. Exercising may feel like a punishment because you may have to work all the hours God has sent for you to lose a substantial amount of weight. At the end of the day, it is worth it because it is the secret to a complete lifestyle change.

When all is said and done, whichever weight loss procedure you choose, if it is safe and fast, it will bring out all the beauty in you for the whole world to see. Well, beauty may be only skin deep, but what else do you want—a great-looking spleen?

LOW CALORIE INTAKE

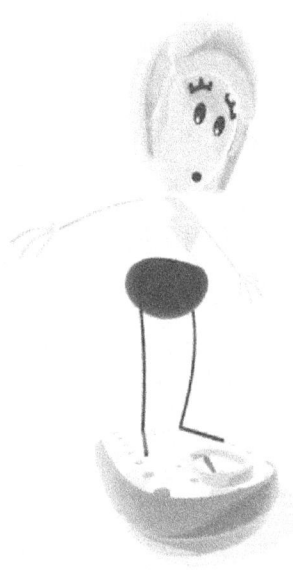

A low-calorie diet is presumably a standout amongst the most well-known approach to shed pounds today. Numerous individuals today stay informed regarding their caloric admission with numerous diverse frameworks. I have seen numerous weight loss organizations advertising this strategy in spite of the fact that it does not generally take an organization to demonstrate to you proper methodologies to do this. You can figure out how to track your calories on your own. Today since everything is more advanced, a number of these calorie counters are electronic based.

A friend of mine even utilizes one on his iPhone. So what is an exceptional ballpark, you ask? Well, a low-calorie eating regimen may as well extend from around 1,200 to 1,500 calories a day. That truly is not a ton of calories; however, it does not fundamentally imply that it is not a great deal of sustenance. You see, you can have bigger parcels of lighter sustenance versus more diminutive partitions of substantial or fattening nourishment.

Assuming that you need to get truly insane you could even strive for a super low-calorie diet. How low? One thousand calories a day. Assuming that you can figure out how to swing that, you are essentially free and will be getting in shape instantly. Presently nobody said that is a simple focus to hit, yet some do. Essentially consuming scraps is all you would be doing assuming that you need to get practical for a moment. Concerning dinners, you truly would not have suppers, and they would be barely sorry excuses for dinners. There are approaches to trap the stomach, however. Consuming something like a rice cake is an outstanding yearning cheat. A rice cake is essentially all air; however, the stomach sees it as an enormous piece of goodness. The issue is that your stomach sees it being something considerable for only so long. When it understands it has been deceived it heads off right once again to snarling and wailing at you.

Therefore, in the event that you are set to do a super-low-calorie diet, just attempt to maintain it for a short period of time. Studies have indicated that most who keep this kind of intense eating methodology going, just keep it going for so long and at any rate move go down to a standard low-calorie eating regimen, having to move down to around 1,400 calories in a day. Getting in shape will come quickly with an amazingly low calorie tally, which is extraordinary! Yet wouldn't it be great if we could be reasonable? You are not set to keep up this pace until the end of time. Making lasting changes to your conducts and propensities with sustenance should not be overlooked. Indeed, that is the support of all weight reduction standards.

Give it a shot and see what you think. It is a month-to-month transformation and does not come immediately overnight. Presently here is one last essential suggestion before I wrap here. Assuming that you're set to attempt this sort of eating regimen, don't think for a moment you can only go out and consume whatever you need exactly as long you stay inside your calorie edge. Generally, exceedingly transformed nourishments with additives and heaps of fats will run up your calorie tally extremely snappy regardless of the fact that it was an exceptionally little segment. This sustenance has a tendency to abandon you with craving and obviously extremely poor dietary worth.

Without fitting supplements and an equalized eating regimen, numerous negative impacts might occur incorporating low vigor, expanded appetite, cerebral pain, tiredness, stress or disposition swings and, obviously, self-regard. You will be much more content with yourself when consuming high supplement and filament sustenance with low calories. It is even conceivable to shed pounds by consuming more nourishment than you were initially. Overall, low-calorie diets work, yet keep some things in mind when consuming the contrast between the great, the awful, and the outright appalling. Here are a few examples.

Crude Fresh Vegetables

Low in calories and high in fiber, vegetables are a perfect hopeful to nibble on. Because of their high fiber content, they help us feel full and are an improved elective to filling snacks like scones or potato chips.

By joining crude vegetables with low-calorie dips, salsa or hummus, we can fulfill our yearning between meals without trading off our calorie admission arrange.

Carrots, broccoli, peppers, cauliflower, tomatoes and celery all possess all the necessary qualities to include crunch and mixed bag, crossing over that hole between meals.

New Fruit

High in fiber and rich in cancer-prevention agents, tree-grown foods are a top-notch, low-calorie nibble. The greater part of us pine for a little sweetness, especially when centered eagerly on our objective, and the common sugars in products of the soil can offer us this without bargaining our eating methodology. Because of their high water content, apples and oranges and, for example, melon, blackberries, raspberries, strawberries, grapefruit, oranges and fruits and in addition various others are exceptionally low in calories.

Assuming that consuming tree grown foods as it is does not request, why not utilize our creative energy and make purees to combine with yogurt to structure an invigorating drink? Pineapple is an astounding decision to blend with bungalow or low-fat cream cheddar. Poached pears or prepared fruits make a filling and agreeable hot sweet treat.

Stuffed Tomatoes or Mushrooms

Tomatoes and mushrooms are both low calorie and flexible. Brisk and simple to get ready, they make a simple nibble, or even in a bigger parcel a fundamental supper.

By joining finely slashed peppers, onions, fish in saline solution and some garlic, we have a wonderful, low-calorie filling for our tomatoes or mushrooms. Add a shower of low-calorie vegetable oil and they are primed to heat.

Other cooked meats or fish can additionally be utilized, or might be made into a veggie lover version, maybe with tofu or a ratatouille sort filling.

Tasty, low in calories, high in fiber and a perfect mid-dinner nibble, we may as well feel managed without being enticed to pass on awful eating propensities.

Assortment and creative energy will all help in the outcomes we can accomplish in our journey to get more fit steadily without feeling eager between suppers. Variety is unquestionably the zest of life concerning low-calorie snacks. We can make countless divine mixes of snacks utilizing fixings that we both like and have a low-calorie check. All we need is a little time and creative ability.

Five Tips to Keep Weight Off After the 1,000-Calorie Diet

1. Eat 5 times each day.

2. Eat every 2 to 3 hours per day every day. This keeps your body in a state of processing.

3. Combining starches, fats and proteins serves to keep away from fat space.

4. If you should consume pasta, dependably consume it in the unanticipated morning or early evening.

5. Cut back on fruit juices and beverage dark espresso, tea and water.

Sound Diet Food Suggestions

You can blend and match these foods and others in your everyday feast plan. These are just a proposal to kick you off.

*Medium golden apple

*Ground turkey

*Eat protein and vegetables

*Lean chicken/turkey

*Extra virgin olive oil to cook with

*Spinach salad/olive oil

*Brown rice (long grain)

*Cooked broccoli

The 1,800-Calorie Diet

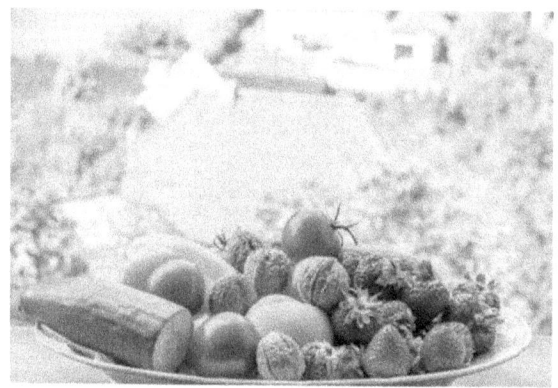

Most people find losing weight by counting their calories to be a hassle. Measuring and sorting food takes time and effort in a day and age when grab-and-go food has become the norm. But studies have proven that if you are conscious of the amount of food you consume daily you are more likely to eat responsibly and lose weight. And not by just a little! Some studies found that people who tracked their nutrition were twice as likely to meet their weight goals. The trick to counting calories is doing it all at once! By pre-planning your meals for the entire day, there is no counting to be done when you are hungry. You can just grab food out of your pre-planned regimen and the thought of counting those calories doesn't even have to cross your mind! Here is an example of a week of delicious and calorie-conscious pre-planned meals:

If there are dietary restrictions or preferences, simply replace them with a similar sized (and calorie) option.

1,800-calorie Sunday:

Breakfast: 300 calories

8 ounces of oatmeal

1 ounce blueberries or strawberries

1 ounce walnuts or almonds

Snack: 200 calories

1 tbsp. peanut butter or almond butter

5 celery sticks or 1 apple

Lunch: 500 calories

5 ounces whole grain pasta

1 ounce pesto sauce

1 chicken breast (4 ounces)

Snack: 200 calories

2 ounces hummus

10 carrot sticks

Dinner: 500 calories

Vegetable Stir Fry

1 ounce teriyaki sauce

4 ounces salmon

Dessert: 100 calories

6 ounces of frozen red grapes

1,800-calorie Monday:

Breakfast: 500 calories

Egg white omelet with peppers, onions

2 slices bacon

2 slices whole wheat toast

Snack: 200 calories

1 cup low-fat yogurt

12 raw almonds

Lunch: 300 calories

Turkey sandwich on whole wheat bread

Slice tomato

Slice cheese

Broccoli sprouts

1 tsp. mustard

Snack: 200 calories

4 ounces salsa

1 ounce tortilla chips

Dinner: 500 calories

4 ounces roast chicken

1 small baked sweet potato

1 pat of butter, cinnamon

1 side salad, 1 tsp. of dressing

Dessert: 100 calories

5 ounce strawberries dusted with

1 tsp. of chocolate powder

1,800-calorie Tuesday:

Breakfast: 300 calories

2 ounces muesli

1 cup low-fat yogurt

Snack: 200 calories

1 apple

1 tbsp. peanut butter

Lunch: 500 calories

Spinach Salad with

4 ounces chicken breast

1 ounce dried cranberries

1 ounce walnuts

1 ounce vinaigrette

Snack: 200 calories

1 ounce pita chips

1 ounce hummus

Dinner: 500 calories

3 ounces of grilled shrimp

6 ounces steamed vegetables

4 ounces steamed wild rice

Dessert:

1 ounce/2 chocolate chip cookies 100 calories

1,800-Calorie Wednesday:

Breakfast: 300 calories

8 ounces of oatmeal

1 ounce blueberries or strawberries

1 ounce walnuts or almonds

Snack: 200 calories

1 ounce cottage cheese

2 slices of pineapple

Lunch: 500 calories

Greek Salad

1 ounce Mediterranean dressing

0.5 ounces olives

2 ounces onion

4 ounces cucumber

2 spicy peppers

3 ounces grilled chicken

Snack: 200 calories

1 ounce pita chips

1 ounce hummus

Dinner: 500 calories

5 ounces whole wheat pasta

2 ounces tomato sauce

2 ounces ground turkey or beef

1 slice wheat bread with olive oil and garlic

Dessert: 100 calories

5 ounces strawberries dusted with

1 tsp. of chocolate powder

1,800-calorie Thursday:

Breakfast: 300 calories

2 ounces muesli

1 cup low fat yogurt

Snack: 200 calories

6 ounces fruit salad

Lunch: 400 calories

Asian Lettuce wraps:

4 ounces ground turkey

0.5 ounce teriyaki sauce

Lettuce leaves for wraps

Snack: 200 calories

1 cup low-fat yogurt

12 raw almonds

Dinner: 600 calories

Eggplant Parmesan (6 ounces)

3 ounces steamed broccoli

Dessert: 100 calories

5 ounces strawberries dusted with

1 tsp. of chocolate powder

1,800-Calorie Friday:

Breakfast: 300 calories

Egg white omelet with peppers, onions

2 slices bacon

Snack: 200 calories

1 ounce cottage cheese

2 slices of pineapple

Lunch: 500 calories

5 ounces whole grain pasta

1 ounce pesto sauce

1 chicken breast (about 4 ounces)

Snack: 200 calories

1 ounce pita chips

1 ounce hummus

Dinner: 500 calories

3 ounces of grilled shrimp

6 ounces steamed vegetables

4 ounces steamed wild rice

Dessert: 100 calories

6 ounces of frozen red or green grapes

1,800-calorie Saturday:

Breakfast: 300 calories

1 slice whole wheat French toast

4 ounces fresh cut fruit

Snack: 200 calories

1 apple

1 tbsp. peanut butter

Lunch: 300 calories

Turkey sandwich on whole wheat bread

Slice tomato

Slice cheese

Broccoli sprouts

1 tsp. mustard

Snack: 200 calories

1 cup low-fat yogurt

12 raw almonds

Dinner: 500 calories

Greek Salad

1 ounce Mediterranean dressing

0.5 ounces olives

2 ounces onion

4 ounces cucumber

2 spicy peppers

3 ounces grilled chicken

Dessert: 100 calories

1 ounce/2 chocolate chip cookies

As you can see, dieting does not mean starving! This is a good amount of food and covers all of the nutrients required for optimal performance. We do not recommend cutting any one nutrient (like carbohydrates or fats) from your diet completely, and we rather suggest that you go with the healthiest of these nutrients when you consume them. An example of this would be whole wheat bread and pasta instead of their bleached counterparts. You can consume healthy fats like the fats in nuts and avocados instead of unhealthy fats in certain prepackaged and fried foods. People tend to eat more food than the suggested servings in general, so this is another way to cut down without eliminating carbs, fats or sugars. Moderation is the key.

How did we get the 1,800-calorie number, you ask? Remember, this is just an example of a calorie counting regimen. The number 1,800 is based on a 25-year-old female's basal metabolic rate. The basal metabolic rate (BMR) is the number of how many calories you need to maintain the weight you are now. To calculate your own personal basal metabolic rate you can consult a nutritionist, personal trainer or use a number of online resources to calculate it for yourself. Once you have your basal metabolic rate you can adjust your calories for weight loss. Be sure to take your activity levels into account; a person who sits all day at work would need fewer calories than a person who walks stairs all day long!

The measurements are based on the weight of the foods rather than the volume. Because of this, it would be in your best interest to invest in a digital kitchen scale. The scale takes the guesswork out of the daily menu planning so that you aren't accidentally consuming more than your chosen servings.

Another helpful tip is to write everything down. It depends on the person, but if you get into the habit of writing your food down you can count your calories much easier. Try using a food journal or creating a calendar with your menu on it and placing it on your fridge. You can even use an app on your smartphone or another online resource. Some online sites have calorie databases to make your calorie counting even more convenient. These websites will even allow you to track calories burned once you decide to integrate fitness into your weight loss regimen. Once you have your calorie counting down to a science, we recommend increasing your activity to burn the calorie candle from both ends, as we like to say.

Losing weight by counting your calories is the most effective way to trim down, but you have to be diligent and accurate using this method. The good news is that once you build the habit into your daily routine, counting calories gets easier with time. Before long you will be an expert at gauging portion sizes and calorie counts. In the meantime, a little pre-planning can go a long way to helping you meet your fitness goals this year!

SET YOUR METABOLISM ON FIRE:

A FAST METABOLISM DIET

We all owe to ourselves a lifestyle of wellness. And a healthier way of eating is the best way to do it. With a fast metabolism diet, you ensure that you make good sense of nutrition. The whole idea is about focusing on eating foods. So you do not have to focus on calorie counting anymore, few or no workouts every day and you can still eat three meals a day, as well as some snacks in between. For anyone seeking to lose weight, it is important to know that planning for your meals is the key to success. Prepped and planned meals should be made the goal, not an option, and that is how you start it going for a fast metabolism diet.

By adopting a fast diet, you opt for a plan that will assist your body to induce physiological changes that set the metabolism on fire. And just like any other weight loss program, there are guidelines; rather, some important facts to note. As you consider this program it should be clear that you have to eat and the more weight you have to lose the more the food you will need to eat to keep that metabolism roaring. Therefore, your first step should be to determine your goal weight. Note that this diet program needs to be conducted in phases for it to work. Through these phases you will have to eat certain portions of foods that will keep you going. Consequently, every portion size is a clear indication of the amount of weight that you wish to lose. And for you to succeed through the fast diet program, you also need to avoid certain foods. They include wheat, and this means you cannot take wheat products such as bread, cereals, crackers, cakes or cookies; the only exception is wheat in sprouted form. You should also avoid corn of all forms, be it corn tortillas, corn chips, grits, hominy or processed foods containing corn. All types of dairy, soy, refined sugar, alcohol, dried fruits and fruit juices, artificial sweeteners and coffee should also be avoided. This in essence will help you eliminate many unhealthy options.

Essentially, a fast metabolism diet is not a miracle—you get to eat real food, in the correct amounts, drink lots of water and maybe exercise a little bit to pull through with it. One of the most successful ways of pulling through with this diet program is by following a three-stage plan that goes for four cycles.

That is, the first phase goes from—preferably—Monday to Tuesday, the second Wednesday to Thursday, while the third takes Friday to Sunday. This then goes on for the next four weeks.

Follow through the plan and eat the recommended portions as I will illustrate in the subsequent paragraphs.

*stage one: the focus should be on carbs and fruits; it would be advisable to start on a Monday to help you follow through with the program. The following meals should be your main focus.

Take 3 carb-rich, low-fat meals with moderate proteins and at least two fruit snacks every day. You should take this 5 times in a day for every 3 to 4 hours. Ensure that you also take enough complex carbohydrates every day.

For your breakfast, you can have grain and fruit—this should be within 30 minutes of waking. Three hours later you can then have a fruit snack.

For lunch, which should be three hours later, some protein, vegetables and fruit can do. Your second fruit snack should come sometime later after your lunch.

Dinner should be more or less the same as lunch, that is, proteins, grains and vegetables.

As I mentioned earlier, fast food metabolism diet requires you to eat. But you eat depending on the amount of weight that you need to lose so this means you have to follow through a certain portion size. So if you intend to lose 20 pounds or less, you can eat appropriate vegetables for any phase. For proteins, you can take four ounces of meat, six ounces of fish or a cup of cooked legumes in all the stages. Only three egg whites should be taken. For grains, you can eat one cup of cooked grains or a cup of pretzels. For fruits, one piece of an appropriate fruit is enough. If you ensure that you maintain this portion size, your metabolism ought to work for your benefit. In case you need to lose some additional 20 pounds, add a half portion to the above portion size. You can bet that this plan works, and by keeping your metabolism guessing in such a specific and deliberate way, you will have it working much faster to give you better results.

*stage two: comes between Wednesday and Thursday. Meals high in protein and high vegetables as well as low fats are recommended. The aim of this phase of fast metabolism diet is to unlock stored fats and build muscles. Your meals should, therefore, include 3 high-protein, low-fat, low-carb snacks and 2 protein snacks. And just as in phase 1, eat 5 times in a day and every 3 to 4 hours. The following program should be followed through from breakfast to dinner.

Breakfast should consist of vegetables and proteins 30 minutes after waking, followed by a protein snack after 3 hours. Lunch will be comprised of proteins and vegetables (3 hours later) followed by a protein snack. Finally for dinner, you should have some more veggies and proteins. You should follow through the portion size indicated above only that in the second phase there should be no consumption of grains.

*stage three: Where you unleash the burn, you should concentrate on healthy fats, moderate carbohydrates, moderate proteins and low glycemic fruits. Your breakfast should consist of fruit, fat or protein, grain and vegetables. Note: the two snacks required for the day should have vegetables, fat or protein. Both lunch and dinner should have vegetables, fat or protein with the option of some grain or starch during dinner. Similarly, in this phase, the portion size is the same as the one indicated for the first phase only that it includes fat consumption.

For fat consumption, one avocado, ¼ cup of raw nuts or seed butter could serve you right.

One thing about the fast metabolism diet is that it is satisfying. It ensures that your body gets quality vitamins and minerals as well as lots of water. In every stage of the fast metabolism diet, consumption of organic foods in encouraged whenever it is possible. Organic produce helps stop preservatives, additives, pesticides, and hormones from slowing the liver as it burns the fat.

A Healthy Start with a Low-Carb Diet

Low-carbohydrate diets used to be a fad, but now there's more and more evidence that such nutritional plans are actually very healthy. Generally speaking, low-carb diets get rid of most grains, certain fats, processed foods and foods in which sugar is added. Meats, fish, eggs and many other foods are recommended, as are vegetables, fruits, and nuts.

There are numerous benefits to low-carbohydrate diet plans. Many of these have been proven over time and others are benefits that people report after changing to a low-carb diet. After considering various positive effects of this type of diet, we'll look at which foods to include and which to avoid, and offer a basic plan that will help you get started on your low-carbohydrate diet.

Proven Effects:

Low-carbohydrate diet plans have been proven to offer the following:

*Weight loss without restricting calories

*Measurable improvement in triglycerides

*Documented reduction in blood glucose for diabetics and pre-diabetics

*An increase in HDL cholesterol (that's the "good" variety)

*Decreased levels in blood insulin

*Better insulin sensitivity

*Reduction in blood pressure

Reported Effects:

Those effects alone make a good case for a low-carb diet. Still, there are other benefits that have been reported by those following low-carbohydrate diet plans. Although not scientifically proven, there is growing evidence to support these claims, and the scientific community has become more interested in these possible positive effects.

Positive Effects:

The following have been reported but not necessarily as consistently noted as those above:

*Increased energy

*Decreased cravings for sweets

*Ability to concentrate more consistently

*Less moodiness and less compulsive behavior

*Better dental health, including fewer gum problems and less plaque

Also, people have noted the following:

*Less joint or muscle pain

*Reduction in number of headaches

*Improvement in PMS, with it being less severe

*Fewer problems with digestion, heartburn, etc.

*Healthier skin

Basics of Low-Carbohydrate Diet Plans

Here are some solid general guidelines regarding what your low-carbohydrate diet plan should consist of and what it should exclude. Natural, organic foods are best. Staying away from foods that have been over-processed is recommended.

Basic Good Foods

*Meat, fish, eggs

*Vegetables, fruit, nuts, seeds

*High-fat dairy

*Fats, healthy oils and possibly tubers and non-gluten grains

Foods Not Recommended:

*Sugar

*High fructose corn syrup

*Wheat

*Seed oils, trans fats

*Artificial sweeteners, "diet" and low-fat products

*Highly processed foods

Foods to avoid:

*Sugar in cereals, ice cream and any processed foods with sugar

*Grains that have gluten, such as wheat, barley and rye

*Hydrogenated or partially hydrogenated oils, that is trans fats

*High Omega-6, seed and vegetable oils, such as sunflower, canola and corn oils

*Artificial sweeteners

*Any diet or low-fat products

*Foods that have been highly processed

Low-Carbohydrate Diet Plan Specifics:

Specifically, there are better types of meats, fish, eggs and other foods to eat. As an example, meats such as beef, lamb, pork, turkey and chicken are all fine, with those that are grass-fed being the best.

Wild fish is better for the consumer than farm-raised, with salmon, trout, haddock, cod, shrimp and many others fitting well within a low-carb diet plan. In terms of eggs, it's been found that Omega-3-enriched or pastured eggs are preferred.

There's a range of great vegetables that you can enjoy, such as spinach, tomatoes, carrots, cauliflower, broccoli and asparagus. Apples, oranges, pears, blueberries and strawberries and various seeds and nuts, such as almonds, walnuts and sunflower seeds, are all a part of a low-carb plan.

Cheese, heavy cream, butter and yogurt are recommended and various fats and oils, such as coconut oil, butter, lard, olive oil and cod fish liver oil are considered to be good.

Preferred drinks include water, coffee, tea and carbonated beverages that don't contain artificial sweeteners.

Diet Plan

One thing about low-carb diets is they are flexible, and you can actually eat a lot on them. Here's a basic plan that you can start with. The point is to get used to cutting down on carbs while enjoying more fresh foods, and those that are prepared in a healthier manner. Use this diet as a starting point and feel free to experiment, while avoiding those foods that should always be avoided.

Monday

Breakfast

Omelet (3 eggs)

Kale and onions prepared in butter or coconut oil

1/2 cup vegetable juice.

Lunch

Grass-fed yogurt (8 ounces)

Blueberries

Handful of almonds

Dinner

Cheeseburger (4 ounces, no bun)

Streamed broccoli and salsa sauce.

Tuesday

Breakfast

3 slices turkey bacon

2 poached eggs

Lunch

Chicken salad sandwich with tomatoes and lettuce wrapped in a low-carb tortilla

Dinner

Baked salmon (6 ounces) with butter and served with steamed asparagus

Wednesday

Breakfast

Rosemary lemon tea

Low-carb waffles

Low-carb maple syrup

Lunch

Shrimp salad (8 ounces)

1 teaspoon olive oil

Kale chips

Dinner

Skinless chicken (6 ounces)

1 cup roasted vegetables with parsley

Thursday

Breakfast

Green tea with mint

3 scrambled eggs

One cup of chopped bell peppers

1 ounce cheese

2 turkey sausage links

Lunch

Smoothie with coconut milk

1 cup berries

A few almonds

Protein powder

Dinner

Steak and steamed cauliflower and broccoli with basil

Friday

Breakfast

Scrambled eggs (3)

Turkey sausage

2 low-carb tortillas

Salsa

Lunch

Chicken salad with some olive oil served with fresh tomatoes, cucumbers, red peppers and onion.

Dinner

2 pork chops seasoned with oregano with parsley spiced baked tomato, onion, green pepper combo (12 ounces)

Saturday

Breakfast

Cheese omelet

Bacon (2 slices)

½ cup of vegetable juice

Lunch

Roast beef salad (5 ounces roast beef) with cheddar cheese (2 ounces), sliced tomatoes and cucumbers and chopped celery drizzled in olive oil

Dinner

Meatballs (5 ounces) with lightly stir-fried Italian peppers, green beans and plum tomatoes flavored with basil and oregano

Sunday

Breakfast

Veggie omelet with 2 turkey sausage links

Lunch

Smoothie with coconut milk (16 ounces), a bit of heavy cream, chocolate-flavored protein powder and berries

Dinner Grilled chicken wings (8 ounces) with raw spinach on the side

Keep It Interesting

The diet plan above utilizes a variety of meats. Be sure to keep things interesting when switching to a low-carb diet plan. Use a wide range of vegetables and be sure to include plenty of fish. Fish is an excellent source of nutrients that aid the body in a variety of ways, and it is also fast to prepare. Thus, if you're a person who says that they don't have time for a new way of eating, add a lot of fish to your diet. It usually takes around 10 minutes to cook. Eggs can also be prepared quickly.

Use spices to make things interesting. Four common spices that are simply fantastic when combined are parsley, basil, oregano and tarragon. Use two, three or all four at a time. Rosemary can also be a great addition to chicken, fish and vegetable dishes. Also, feel free to utilize various cheeses, as these are highly recommended for low-carb diets. Swiss, various forms of cheddar, Muenster and Monterey jack cheese make fine additions to eggs, vegetable dishes and sandwiches.

Changing For the Better

Many people have found that low-carbohydrate diet plans have changed how they feel and have improved their mental and physical health. There is a lot to recommend in going low carb, and it's not difficult at all to make the switch. Add to the diet some exercise, and you're on your way to a whole new healthier you.

THE PALEO DIET

The Paleo diet is known as 'The Caveman Diet' for a good reason. It has one rule and one rule only: if a caveman couldn't eat it then, you can't eat it now.

So, what does this mean? It means you are allowed to eat anything that could have been hunted or gathered during the Paleolithic era (hence the name Paleo diet). This includes any kind of meat, fish, seeds, eggs, regional vegetables, nuts and leafy greens. Anything processed such as Pop Tarts, frozen pizzas and ice cream have to go! Also, anything containing wheat or wheat gluten is not allowed. Instead of filling your body with these nutrient-deficient foods, you will be fueling it with nutrient dense ones.

Why should I follow a diet used by cavemen? Didn't they have short lifespans? Yes. Their lifespans were much shorter than ours due to enduring extreme weather and the dangers of having to hunt for their food in the wild. If they had the modern day conveniences of shelter, heat and air-conditioning we have, their lifespan would have far surpassed ours.

One of the main benefits of following the Paleo lifestyle is the fact that you can put away the calorie counters and food scales. Because you are eating whole, nutrient dense foods that your body can burn as fuel, you may eat until you are full without worrying about portion sizes or calorie counting. You eat only when you are hungry. If you are hungry only twice a day, then eat twice a day. If you are hungry every four hours, then so be it. Only eat when you are hungry and only eat until you are full, not stuffed.

Worried that not counting calories or measuring portions will lead to weight gain? Don't be! Because the Paleo diet is low in carbohydrates, it forces the body into a state of ketosis, which burns fat for energy instead of glycogen. Glycogen (glucose) is prevalent in the body when a person consumes too many carbohydrate-laden foods such as cakes, pies and bread. Being in a state of ketosis causes you to have a constant stream of energy and a lean, muscular body.

How can eating a low-carb diet full of meat and eggs be healthy? Don't we need fiber? Fiber is essential for our body to function correctly and the Paleo diet is full of fiber in the form of vegetables and fruits. This is a low-carb lifestyle, but is NOT to be confused with other low-carb diets such as Atkins. Whereas diets of that type are extremely restrictive when it comes to carbohydrates, the Paleo lifestyle allows moderate amounts that come from plant-based sources.

Now that you know what the Paleo diet is, let's get to the good part: the food. You may think this lifestyle is pretty restrictive given the short list of acceptable foods mentioned above. Actually, there are hundreds, if not thousands, of tasty Paleo-friendly recipes out there. A quick internet search will point you to pages of Paleo diet cookbooks, recipes and blogs. There are recipes available for all levels of cooking skills, from the insanely simple three-ingredient Paleo pancake to the more elaborate four-course dinner.

Below you will find an entire week's worth of Paleo-friendly meals, just to show you how varied and exciting the Paleo lifestyle can be. Please keep in mind that there is no measuring portions. Simply eat until you are comfortably full.

Monday

Breakfast

Loaded Breakfast Hash: A combination of sweet potatoes, green peppers, onions, spinach tomatoes and chicken sausage

Lunch

Zoodles and Meatballs: Zoodles are made by peeling a zucchini with a julienne peeler then topping with meatballs and pasta sauce

Dinner

Pulled Pork Barbecue: A pork shoulder that has been coated with a delicious Ancho chili rub, then slow cooked in a cider vinegar based sauce. Serve with a carrot/parsnip puree.

Tuesday

Breakfast

Green Monster Smoothie: A delicious blend of spinach, kale, banana, pineapple and coconut milk

Lunch

A large salad topped with your favorite meat, nuts, seeds, eggs and avocado

Dinner

Beef Brisket with Peppers: A juicy beef brisket, slow cooked with onions and a variety of peppers. Serve with a large side salad, topped with avocado, nuts, seeds, chopped boiled egg and your choice of vegetables.

Wednesday

Breakfast

Egg Muffins: Wonderful little muffins made with eggs, onions and peppers

Lunch

Chicken Salad: A hearty chicken salad served on a bed of lettuce

Dinner

Garlic and Herb Crusted Pork Loin: A tender pork loin coated with a mix of crushed garlic and fresh herbs, then roasted in the oven. Serve with shredded apple coleslaw.

Thursday

Breakfast

Breakfast Burrito: Egg whites and your choice of chopped vegetables rolled up in a slice of ham

Lunch

Raw Vegetable Platter: A filling plate of your choice of vegetables with a side of avocado dip

Dinner:

Salmon with Lemon Dill Sauce: A thick cut of wild caught salmon, smothered in a tangy lemon dill sauce. Serve with roasted broccoli.

Friday

Breakfast

Cinnamon Raisin Bread: Paleo friendly bread? Yes! You can bake up a moist, flavorful bread with almond flour, raw honey and juicy raisins.

Lunch

Chicken Wraps: Strips of grilled chicken and peppers, wrapped in lettuce leaves

Dinner

Chicken Pot Pie: A creamy chicken pot pie topped with a crunchy, almond flour crust. Serve with a side salad.

Saturday

Breakfast

Coconut Flour Waffles: Warm, fluffy waffles made with coconut flour, raisins and cinnamon

Lunch

Lamb Burgers: Tender, juicy lamb burgers topped with fresh mint and wrapped in lettuce leaves

Dinner

Crispy Chicken and Cauliflower: Flavorful, crispy chicken thighs served with mashed cauliflower

Sunday

Breakfast

Breakfast Scramble and Biscuits: Eggs scrambled with your choice of fresh vegetables, served with almond flour biscuits

Lunch

Shrimp Scampi: Tasty shrimp cooked in a zesty lemon pepper sauce

Dinner

Crispy Orange Duck: A slow-roasted duck breast, smothered in a sweet orange sauce. Serve with steamed carrots.

As you can see, the Paleo diet is anything but restrictive. With such a wide variety of delicious meals to choose from, there is no reason for you to not live a Paleo lifestyle. Simply try it for 30 days. Your skin will be clearer, your belly less bloated and your energy levels higher. Your entire body will thank you.

GLUTEN-FREE DIET

One of the most popular diets in the current times is the gluten-free diet. Gluten is a protein that is present in wheat related grains such as foods containing barley, rye, wheat, oats, and malt. It also is a protein often added to give foods flavor and in many processed foods. Basically it refers to the protein that is present in almost all of our staple food products like cereals, bread, pasta and desserts. Gluten is one of the most essential components of traditionally baked products, as this gives the fluffy and moist texture of the muffins and cakes. Other sources of gluten are soy sauce, beer, salad dressings and processed cheese. A gluten-free diet facilitates weight loss when consumption of the glutinous carbohydrates is completely stopped and substituted by superior quality and nutritious food.

Following a gluten-free diet is not only fun and easy but it is also extremely effective. One can expect to lose a minimum of two pounds per week by following a gluten-free diet by consuming a diet that is of 1,500 calories per day instead of 2,200 calories, which is the nutritional count of an average diet followed by Americans. Below is a detailed weekly meal plan of a gluten-free diet. The plan recommends eating 2-3 meals a day with additional veggies and fruits included in the diet. This gluten-free diet plan coupled with light exercises is undoubtedly going to help you shed the unwanted pounds.

Monday

Breakfast

Tofu scrambled - 2 cups

Tangerine - 1

Zero calorie beverage or tea - 1 cup

Lunch

Brown rice and vegetables - 3 cups

Carrots cut in the form of sticks - 1 cup with 1 tsp. salad dressing

Snack

Almonds - 1/2 ounce

Raisins - 2 tbsp.

Dinner

Rice macaroni and cheese - 1 cup

Mixed green vegetables - 1 1/2 cups

Vinegar - 1 tbsp.

Dessert

Peaches (fresh or frozen) - ½ cup

*Nutritional components of this meal

Protein - 41 grams

Calories - 1,290

Fat - 60 grams

Sodium - 2,055

Carbohydrates - 159

Fiber - 24 grams

Tuesday

Breakfast

1 1/2 cups of gluten free cereal

1/2 cup of soy milk

1/2 tsp. cinnamon

Snack

1 apple

1 ounce string cheese

Lunch

1 bowl of cream and tomato soup

1 1/2 cups mixed green salad

Snack

1 cup low-fat yogurt

1/2 cup juice of a freshly crushed pineapple

Dinner

Shepherd's pie

1 piece bread which is essentially gluten-free

1 cup boiled broccoli garnished with half ounce of grated parmesan cheese

Dessert

1 small pear

1/2 cup plain yogurt flavored with vanilla extract

*Nutritional components of this meal

Protein - 2 ounces

Calories - 1,423

Fat - 1.5 ounces

Sodium - 2,922

Carbohydrates - 200

Fiber - 1 1/2 ounces

Wednesday

Breakfast

Mexican scrambled tofu

4 ounces of orange juice

Lunch

2 brown rice cakes and 1 cup of boiled vegetables

2 sliced stalks of celery

1/2 cup of cucumber cut in the shape of sticks

1 tbsp. of salad dressing on the celery and cucumber salad

Snack

1 tbsp. almond butter

2 rice cakes

Dinner

Cheese Mexican Enchilada - 3 pieces

3 cups of spinach leaves tossed with 2 tsp. of salad dressing.

Dessert

1 cup low-fat milk

1/2 cup frozen strawberries

*Nutritional components of this meal

Protein - 1 ½ ounces

Calories - 1,415

Fat - 1 ounce

Sodium - 2,551

Carbohydrates - 159

Fiber - 1 ounce

Thursday

Breakfast

1.5 ounce of organic cream and rice

1 cup low-fat yogurt with one small pear

Lunch

2 cups of black bean vegetable soup garnished with one ounce of grated low-fat cheese

1/2 cup diced cucumber

Snack

1 cup cottage cheese

1/2 cup blueberries

Dinner

4 ounces macaroni and cheese

1 ½ cups of mixed green veggies dressed in 1 tbsp. of vinegar

*Nutritional components of this meal:

Protein - 3 ounces

Calories - 1,320

Fat - 1 ounce

Sodium - 2,446

Carbohydrates - 196

Fiber - 1 ounce

Friday

Breakfast

1.5 ounces Mexican scrambled tofu

1/2 cup pineapple and 1 cup low-fat milk blended into a smoothie

Lunch

2 cups rice soup and organic beans

1 slice of bread

2 cups of green salad dressed with one tbsp. of salad dressing and 2 tsp. of sunflower seeds

Snack

Half cup sticks of celery

Dinner

1 bowl of Indian vegetable curry

1 corn tortilla

1 bowl of raita (this is cucumber, tomato, onion and chili sliced into small pieced and combined with low fat yogurt)

*Nutritional components of this meal:

Protein - 2 ounces

Calories - 1,326

Fat - 2 ounces

Sodium - 2,450

Carbohydrates - 191

Fiber - 24 grams

Saturday

Breakfast

1 1/2 tsp. of raisins

1 apple

1 slice toasted bread (gluten free)

1 cup low-fat soy milk

Lunch

1 cup vegetable curry with organic chili

3 cups of green salad dressed with light salad dressing

Snack

1/2 ounce of sunflower seeds

2 tbsp. raisins

Dinner

Roasted vegetable soup garnished with 2 tbsp. of grated parmesan cheese

1 slice toasted bread

2 cups of salad dressed with one tbsp. vinegar and 2 tsp. extra virgin olive oil

Dessert

1 cup fruit (either frozen or fresh)

*Nutritional components of this meal:

Protein - 51 grams

Calories - 1,479

Fat - 46 grams

Sodium - 1,990

Carbohydrates - 227

Fiber - 31 grams

Sunday

Breakfast

1 cup nonfat yogurt with one cup frozen berries

1/2 cereal (gluten free)

2 tsp. of almonds

Lunch

2 cups of tomato soup with cream

2 cups green salad

4 gluten-free crackers

Snack

1/2 ounce of cashew nuts (raw)

1 tbsp. raisins

Dinner

Mexican whole bean enchilada

2 cups of spinach

1 tbsp. sesame seeds dressed with two tbsp. of lime juice and one tsp. of olive oil

*Nutritional components of this meal:

Protein - 46 grams

Calories - 1,310

Fat - 49 grams

Sodium - 2,220

Carbohydrates - 195

Fiber - 27 grams

This is a very effective meal plan which helps to shed the extra pounds. It is also possible that you can even add variation to this diet by substituting the above mentioned fruits and vegetables with other gluten-free foods. Below is a list of gluten-free foods that will be of immense help to people who intend to follow a gluten-free diet. It is important to note that all fruits and vegetables are gluten-free in their natural state. Even meats are gluten free if they are unprocessed and not fried. The types of meat which are gluten free are beef, chicken, duck, lamb, goose, venison, pork, rabbit and turkey.

Dairy products which are gluten free are eggs, cheese, cream, sour cream, yogurt and low-fat milk. The most important foods which people have a lot of confusion about are grains, flour and wheat. The ones which are allowed in a gluten-free diet and are commonly used are: almond flour, bean flour, corn flour, soy flour, potato flour, brown rice, corn meal, corn starch, rice, polenta, flax seed and tapioca. Other gluten-free foods include baking soda, honey, jam, nuts, oil, most spices, juice, vinegar and wine.

Now that we have listed all the gluten-free foods, following are some of the gluten-free recipes that are not only healthy but extremely tasty. The first dish is a main course that is slow-cooked pork belly along with stir-fried rice with egg. What is important to note here is that the rice should just be stir-fried and not fried excessively because it will not remain gluten free. Stir-fried rice is a method where the rice is just tossed in the wok for a few seconds so that all the excess moisture is lost.

*Ingredients required for the pork

1 pound pork belly (boneless along with rind)

Sea salt - 4 tbsp.

Roasted peppercorns (ground) - 2 tbsp.

White pepper - 2 tsp.

Five-spice powder - 2 tbsp.

Caster sugar - 1 tbsp.

Ingredients for the stir-fried rice

Long-grain rice - half kg

Eggs (beaten) - 2

Sesame oil - 2 tsp.

Salt - 1 tsp.

Vegetable or groundnut oil - 2 tbsp.

Black pepper - 1/2 tsp.

Finely chopped spring onions - 2 tbsp.

Preparation

For marinating the pork, take a sharp fork and pierce the rind side so that the skin gets covered with small insertions. Insert a meat hook into the pork and hang it such that the meat can be treated and marinated properly.

In a big pan boil water and pour this boiling water over the rind of the pork a number of times.

Heat a wok and dry roast the pepper, salt, five spice powder and sugar for approximately three minutes.

After the mixture cools down rub the spice mix on the rind of the pork and let the meat hang overnight. This allows the spice mix to get infused with the meat.

While cooking first the oven needs to be preheated to 200' C. Then the pork is placed on a deep roasting pan which is filled with one third part of water. The meat needs to be roasted for 20 minutes.

The next step is to reduce the temperature of the oven to 180' C and let the rind slow cook for two hours. Finally on the last stage the heat is again increased to 230' C where the pork is cooked for 15 minutes and then removed from the oven.

For the fried rice, sesame oil, eggs and a pinch of the salt needs to be mixed on a bowl and kept aside.

Next a large frying pan is kept over heat until it is hot. Add the vegetable oil and then the cooked rice on this wok.

Finally the egg mixture needs to be drizzled over the rice and continued to stir fry till the eggs get cooked. Finally add spring onions, pepper and salt to the rice.

This dish is served along with the slow-cooked pork that is cut into bite size pieces.

The next gluten-free recipe is an amazing salad which not only has multiple components and textures but is also extremely healthy.

Mozzarella and Beetroot salad accompanied with meringues

Ingredients for the meringues

4 egg whites

Caster sugar 250 grams

1/2 ml of beetroot juice

Ingredients for pickled beetroot

Beetroots - 4

Caster sugar - 200 grams

Vinegar - 200 ml

Pinch of salt

Thinly sliced shallots - 2

For beetroot purée

Beetroot juice - 400 ml

Black pepper and salt

Xanthan gum - 1/2 tsp.

Garnish

Cream cheese

Mozzarella

Watercress leaves

Chervil leaves

Preparation

For the meringues, the oven needs to be preheated to 150 degrees and baking trays need to be lined with silicone mats.

In a large food processor the egg whites needs to be whisked until they attain a stiff consistency.

While whisking slowly add the sugar into the meringue until it gets completely folded into the mixture and gets a glossy texture. The beetroot juice is also added one spoon at a time until the mixture gets a pink hue.

Half of the meringue then needs to be filled into a piping bag and the other half needs to be carefully spread over the baking tray with the help of a knife. On the second baking tray pipe out the tiny meringues and bake both the trays for three hours.

To prepare the pickled beetroot, the beetroots need to be placed in a saucepan and covered with water and they need to be boiled until they get tender.

Once the beetroots are cooled enough they need to be peeled and cut into quarters.

Place the sugar, rice wine vinegar and salt in a saucepan and boil them. After removing from the heat, add the cooked beetroots and sliced shallot and set aside until needed.

To prepare the beetroot purée, the beetroot juice is placed in a pan and seasoned with salt and black pepper. The Xanthan gum is then added and the mixture is whisked until it becomes thicker.

To serve, a pastry brush is used to brush the purée on the plates.

Then all the components like the meringues, mozzarella and the pickled beetroot are added to the plate.

Finally the dish is garnished with the watercress and chervil leaves.

Chocolate chip cookies

Ingredients

Cocoa powder - 1 tbsp.

Almond flour - 1 cup

Baking soda - 1/4 tsp.

Sea salt - ¼ teaspoon

3 eggs (both the yolk and the egg whites)

Cinnamon powder - 1/4 tsp.

Vanilla extract - 1/2 tsp.

Honey - 2 tbsp.

Dates -7

Dark chocolate chips -3 tbsp.

Coconut oil - 1/3 of a cup

1 tsp. of avocado oil (this is required to grease the pan)

Procedure

The oven has to be pre-heated to a temperature of 350 degrees.

The baking pan has to be greased with avocado oil and kept aside.

In a food processor the dates, coconut oil, vanilla extract and the two whole eggs are whisked until the ingredients form a smooth paste.

Then dry ingredients, namely flour, baking soda, powdered cinnamon and salt are mixed properly in a mixing bowl.

The egg, dates, vanilla extract and coconut oil paste mixture is added in to these dry ingredients and folded together.

The chocolate chips are added to this mixture.

Finally this mixture is poured into the baking tray already greased with avocado oil and then put in the preheated oven for baking for a minimum 25 minutes.

The gluten-free cookies are ready to be served. This can either be served alone or can be served with the following gluten-free ice cream.

Vanilla Ice cream

Ingredients

Low fat coconut milk - 14.5 ounces

Coconut cream - 1 cup

Vanilla extract - 2 tbsp.

Honey - 2 tbsp.

A pinch of sea salt

1/3 cup unsweetened butter

Procedure

Take the coconut milk, cream, vanilla extract, salt and honey and blend them together in a blender until the mixture becomes a smooth paste.

Turn the ice cream maker on, and on the freezing container pour the blended mixture along with the butter and keep the ice cream maker on until the correct consistency is obtained.

To make the ice cream attain a more firm texture you can refrigerate it for some time. Finally serve this with the chocolate chip cookies and garnish it with roughly chopped hazel nuts.

You can enjoy these two gluten-free dessert recipes either together or individually to your heart's content without having to worry about your health. Hence it can be clearly seen that following a gluten-free diet is not at all difficult. Moreover if cooked with the right mix of ingredients, a gluten-free diet can also be extremely tasty.

The Juice Purge Diet:

Juicing it your way

Juices made from vegetables and fruits are much the same as any sort of sustenance these days. Those days when juices were viewed as substitutes for water are long gone. These were acclimated to extinguish thirst as a sort of hydration. However, these days we find that squeezes are much of the time utilized in addition to going on an eating methodology. Really, the juice scrub has transformed into a comprehensively utilized sort of eating regimen, on the grounds that some respect it to have an edge over different eats less, because of arrangement.

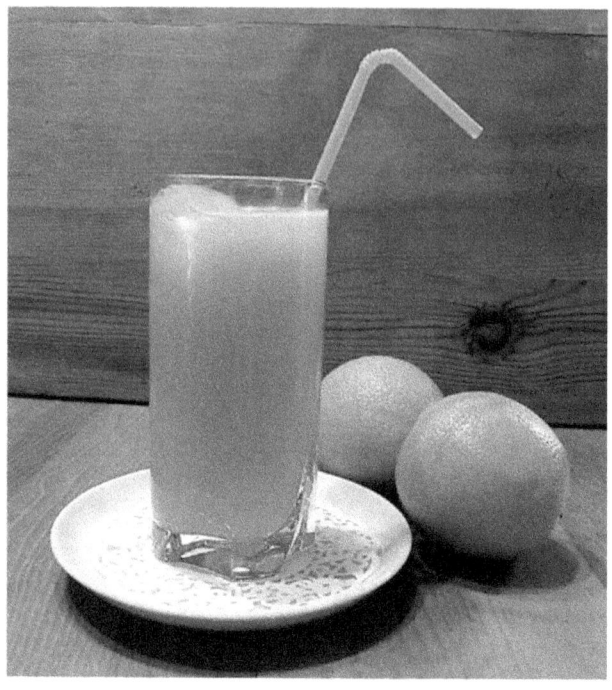

Bunches of individuals who don't especially like products of the soil or veggies find they have the ability to endure the juices a considerable measure all the more effectively. Juice detox is viewed as an eating methodology in fluid structure, made up of the macerated or squashed parts of a product of the soil, or maybe a vegetable. Fruits, red grapes, carrots, celery, kale, cabbage green spinach and tomatoes and, in addition, different vegetables might be the most generally utilized as a part of squeezed eating methodologies. Moreover, the juice wash down is a functional wellspring of vitamins, minerals and hostile to oxidants.

Since we all need a solid approach to lessen our weights, it is no big surprise that one of the every now and again made inquiries today is the sort of apples and oranges that help you shed pounds. In spite of the fact that it may absolutely weigh you down a little when you are simply beginning, incorporating products of the soil in your everyday eating regimen may end up being your redeeming quality in the matter of getting more fit and getting a sound form. When you get the substance of it, it will really turn into second nature to you. The accompanying are the sort of foods grown from the ground you can take assuming that you are intrigued by diminishing your weight the sound way.

The juice purge is a sort of detox program that suggests going on an eating regimen depending only on the admission of squashed veggies or apples and oranges, while completely refusing strong nourishments. Thus, the juice washes down eating.

Methodology might as well basically be utilized for concise measures of time. The standard time of a juice purge is between one and three days, and anything longer than this includes restorative screening for safe results.

Why is juicing so favorable for our general health? Leafy foods juices are incredible for acquiring nourishment and vitamins. Besides, they're less demanding processed than strong sustenance, with the less exacerbation toward the digestive tract. Also because of its profits, the juice furnishes the figure its required opportunity to dispose of destructive poisons without engrossing fresh out of the plastic new ones. Thus, it empowers the liver to have sufficient energy for invigorating and repairing.

All around a juice purify, the form becomes totally detoxified. This purify furnishes the cells and organs inside your physique a chance to quickly dispense with the unsafe poisons you've collected, without retaining fresh out of the plastic new ones concurrently.

Juice detoxifying routines could be incredible for the form, if carried out accurately and never utilized abusively, for instance an accident diet. For a great deal of individuals, squeeze detoxifying techniques are a simple approach to start a healthier living style, while endeavoring to thin down. All around a juice wash down, you'll have the capacity to drop weight quickly, also that you will improve your inside and out health. This works particularly well, assuming that you are utilizing a legitimate vegetable and products of the soil purify system all around the technique. Most variants of juice purify diets incorporates wholesome components. These mixes might additionally be improved utilizing various supplements, for example, zeolite, silica or fundamental olive oil.

An alternate advantage that numerous individuals get from utilizing squeeze detox eating methodologies is expanding in vigor. It's truly an invigorating strategy that can give your physique numerous vitamins, hostile to oxidants, notwithstanding various different components that may enhance your imperativeness and invulnerability. A few juices could even hold proteins that will aid with digestive health as well.

Individuals enthusiastic to get thinner frequently go on low-calorie juice diets and eat fewer carbs. Though a squeeze gives numerous supplements, one needs to consolidate it with some practice administration to lose that weight.

Vegetable juice and apple and orange juices give the form of vitamins and minerals and are needed for solid safety. Vegetable juice can act as ravenousness suppressants and the sugar substance is lower than in soil grown foods juices.

Some low-calorie juice formulas for weight reduction are as follows:

1. Thin Me Juice:

Fixings:

4-5 carrots, half beets

1 celery stalk

1 piece of fruit

Half cucumber

Wash, peel and hack the vegetables and mix in a juicer. You might include ginger assuming that you require some zest in your solid juice!

2. Grapefruit Orange Juice Recipe:

Fixings:

1 grapefruit

3 oranges

Take out the juice of these products of the soil using a blender. Include ice and sample! Grapefruits are helpful for getting in shape. This sound juice is likewise high in vitamin C.

3. 6 ounces Juice (Apple Carrot Celery):

Fixings:

2-3 pieces of fruit

2 carrots

2 celery stalks

2 tbsp. lemon juice

Core the pieces of fruit, peel and cut carrots. Include fruits, carrots, celery and lemon squeeze to a blender and mix well. Spill in glass and include ice if sought. This is a reviving and tasty low-calorie juice.

4. Purging Veggie Broth:

Fixings:

2-3 carrots

2 celery stalks

2 beets

3 kale leaves

1 turnip

Half spinach cluster

Half cabbage head

Half onion

¼ parsley group

2-3 garlic cloves

Boil the above elements and sample! This solid juice will help in detoxification of the figure as well.

5. Papaya Passion Juice:

Fixings:

1 papaya

1 piece of fruit

4-5 dates

Pit the dates and afterward mix all the above parts in a blender. Best when served crisp. This is a solid juice formula.

6. Morning Sunshine Juice:

Fixings:

2 oranges

1 grapefruit

5-6 strawberries

Half banana

Take out the juice from orange and grapefruit. Pour this in the blender with banana and strawberries. Mix well and serve.

7. Carrot Beet juice:

Fixings:

7-8 carrots

Half bubbled and peeled beetroot

4 leaves lettuce

Blend all the elements and revel in this solid juice formula.

Of course, there are many combinations of juicing, either to lose weight or keep healthy. Here are a few more examples.

Green lemonade/green machine:

You will need 2 cups of spinach, 5 kale leaves, 3 stalks of celery, 1 cucumber and a minute piece of ginger.

Directions:

Process all ingredients in a blender, stir or shake and serve.

Benefits:

Weight loss:

Studies conducted by Brazilian nutritionists postulate that the green lemonade has immense benefits. It found out that people who ate two pears or even apples lost more while dieting than those who did not consume any fruit while dieting. Adding a lemon twist to the shake aids in speeding up weight loss. One of the primary benefits of including kale in your juice shake is because it provides a punch with the fewest calories count per class than any other greens. This is probably the most popular of all juicing recipes.

Lower blood pressure:

Similarly, a recent publication by the *Journal of American Nutritionists* suggested that drinking lemon juice is helpful for individuals suffering with cardiovascular problems as it contains potassium. It regulates blood pressure, nausea and dizziness.

Beet:

You will require 5 carrots, 3 medium apples, 4 medium carrots and 1 beet root.

Directions:

Process all ingredients in a juicer, shake and serve.

Benefits:

Liver cleanse:

This undoubtedly is one of the best liver cleansers of all the juicing recipes. The cleansing nature of beets juice is very healing to the liver and bile. Ailments such as hepatitis and jaundice can be reversed.

Colon cancer aversion

Research shows that the pectin in apples or pears lowers the risk of colon cancer by close to 43% and helps maintain a healthy digestive system.

Lower cholesterol:

In addition, the pectin in apples lowers the cholesterol levels. Eating two apples per day may lower the cholesterol level by as much as 18%. Also, ginger reduces the amount of cholesterol absorbed.

Improving eyesight:

Carrots contain vitamin A, whose deficiency can lead to difficulty in seeing in dim-lighted rooms. Since the beet juice recipe contains a lot of carrots, it may keep you away from the ophthalmologist.

Sunset punch:

You will need 2 medium-sized golden delicious apples, 2 large carrots, 2 oranges, 1 sweet red pepper, 1 beet root and 1 sweet potato.

Directions:

Process all ingredients in a juicer, shake and serve.

Benefits:

Aids in stomach cancer prevention

In ancient Greek, beet root was used as a treatment for leukemia. Beet roots contain beta, which belongs to the amino acid class which contains anti-cancer properties. Red beet therapy, which usually entails consumption of close to 3 pounds of raw, mashed beets daily, has been proven to inhibit development of stomach and colon cancers.

Aids digestion:

Apple has a natural laxative. When juiced, apple aids bowel movement due to its gel fiber, pectin that improves the digestive tract ability to expend waste through the gastrointestinal tract.

Enhanced skin complexion:

Carrot juice contains high quality Vitamin C that efficiently replenishes the skin preventing dry skin and other skin blemishes. In addition, orange juice poses anti-oxidant properties that protect the skin from signs of aging.

FAT-FIGHTING SUPER FOODS

When it comes to losing weight, it goes without saying that diet is of the essence. But what really gives it a perfect touch, what makes the difference, is eating foods that burn your fat so fast that you lose weight in a matter of days. What I am here for is to help you know exactly what kind of food helps you achieve that. I am going to go deep, so brace yourself! You may not have been able to succeed in losing weight by other means, but I guarantee you this will work. Everybody tells you the food you should not be eating, but nobody tells you the food you should be eating. That is where I come in. So, start planning how you will get money to buy a couple of new, smaller-sized clothes!

Inflammation is a major cause of obesity. It arises mainly from stress and foods we eat like red meat and trans fats. Now there is a hormone in the body called lepton. This hormone controls appetite and metabolism. When body fat increases, lepton levels increase in the blood, signaling the brain to increase body metabolism and reduce appetite, hence reducing further accumulation of fats. Inflammation interferes with lepton levels in the blood causing the body not to respond to fat levels. That might be the reason why you exercise every day but your body is too stubborn to let go of the fats! Almonds, apples, salmon, bell peppers and egg whites, are natural forms of ibuprofen that stop inflammation. According to research, people who have eaten these have lost as much as a hundred pounds in a span of days! Isn't that something?

Fish is one of the best protein sources. Research shows it is more satisfying than beef or chicken, perhaps because of the types of proteins it contains. Fish is low in fat and rich in omega-3 fatty acids. Omega-3 found in salmon and other fatty fish helps keep fat levels down in one's body. Just ignore the smell; after all, that is a small price to pay for something as big as losing weight, isn't it?

Some foods can help speed up breaking down of fats in your body. Lean meat is one of them. Researchers have proven that including lean meat in your diet helps you burn 5%more kilojoules per day. It takes more energy to digest proteins. The body has to use its fat reserves to provide energy to digest the proteins. Another advantage of lean meat is that it leaves you feeling satisfied and therefore preventing instances of you trying to over-eat later. This is because protein takes a longer time in the stomach. Eating chicken or turkey will do.

Vitamin C is vital too in burning fats. It increases metabolism rates, keeps cholesterol levels in check, and helps dilute fats. A good source of vitamin C is berries, citrus fruits and oranges. Research has proven that taking strawberries before exercise helps burn up 30% more fat. These fruits also help you feel satisfied even after eating little food, due to the large amounts of soluble fiber that take longer to digest. Watermelon, being high in water content, takes up more room in the stomach, hence signaling the body that you're satisfied and don't have space for more. This makes you to take a small amount of food hence less calories. Funny how the body can be manipulated so easily, right?

Calcium is of essence when it comes to losing weight. Eating 1,300 milligrams of calcium a day helps a person lose twice as much weight. Calcium breaks down fat cells and reduces the rate of development of new ones. Low-fat yogurt, cheese or low-fat milk can be good sources of calcium. Apples and pears are also high in water content as well as fiber content, especially if you eat them with peels.

Chickpeas, soybeans and lentils are high in fiber, low in fat and have a low glycemic index, and are therefore effective in weight reduction. Also, soybeans contain a chemical choline, which helps remove fat from the liver. Beans also fall in this category. They are a protein, a vegetable and a great source of fiber, ensuring you stay full at the price of a very small amount of calories. Raw vegetables can help too. They are an amazing snack that satisfies the desire to eat. The water in them helps you feel full, and at the same time is low in calories

Plant-based fats and oily fish contain essential fatty acids that help in burning fat. Adding walnuts or almonds to your diet daily helps to reduce body fat and insulin levels. Fish has been found to reduce women's lepton levels. Salmons, nuts, avocado and flaxseed also do the trick.

Green tea promotes weight loss by stimulating the burning of abdominal fat. It contains catechins, a phytochemical that speeds up the metabolism. Taking hot tea makes it take longer to drink, hence slowing down calorie intake. Cinnamon can be added to the tea too to increase its effectiveness. It boosts sugar metabolism, hence lowering blood sugar levels and helping your body to store less fat. Add some into your tea, or even coffee or yogurt and you will be good to go. Coffee stimulates body metabolism too, hence increasing the rate of losing weight.

Quinoa is another fat-fighting food. It is a type of whole grain food that is easy to cook, satisfies your hunger and is packed with nutrients besides toning down your body fat. Oatmeal also has almost the same benefits but has an added advantage of supplying lots of water to the body. There is a huge importance in taking meals while they are hot. Oatmeal is no exception. Hot food takes a longer time to eat, and all that liquid and the fiber helps you feel full for a longer period.

Another way to fill up your stomach is by eating salad. Lettuce has a high water content that leaves less room in the stomach for fattier foods that you might want to eat. Include a variety of fruits in your salad, but be careful about the dressing; it can add a lot of calories. Dressing your salad with vinegar may help. Vinegar helps burn down fat and at the same time has no calories.

Just as an extra tip, I am going to share a little bit about some spices that can be of great help. Research has proven that people who eat spicy foods consume fewer carbohydrates than the rest. Also, they have a chemical called Capsaicin that triggers thermodynamic burn and speeds up heart rate. The net effect is that more fat is burned. Another interesting spice is turmeric. Turmeric slows down the rate at which fat tissue spreads in animals and lowers triglyceride, blood glucose, fatty acid and cholesterol levels in the body.

Now, start planning which shop to buy clothes from, because you will need a new set in a few weeks' time! And start planning how you will explain to your friends the sudden weight loss!

CHOOSING THE RIGHT EXERCISE PROGRAM

Of all the things we can do for our health, few are more generally helpful than physical exercise. Exercise is vital for good health. Just as we make the time for eating and sleeping, it is vital that we also make the time to remain physically active.

Exercise boosts your immune system and releases brain chemicals that calm you. At the same time, it can increase your fun.

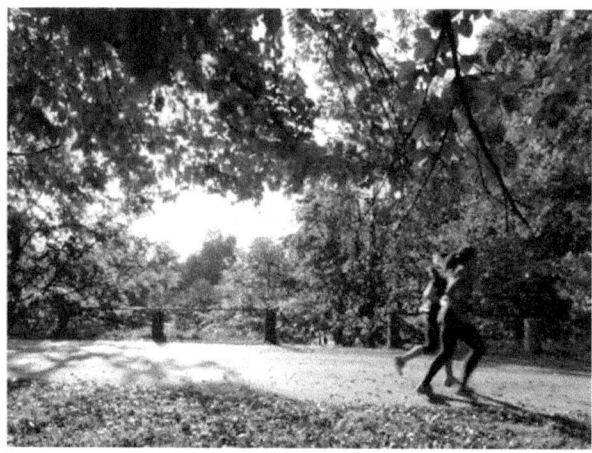

Studies showed that those who exercised regularly also seemed more emotionally stable and less neurotic, they became more organized, and their ability of logical reasoning increased. Persons who get needed exercise sleep better and work better.

But besides simply making one feel better, regular exercise can actually make one healthier and hence more productive. It can even lengthen one's life.

Regular exercise is said to improve the work capacity of the lungs, increases the strength of the heart muscles and halts the loss of lean muscle. Blood circulation and overall health are improved because more oxygen is delivered to body cells. It slows, stops and even reverses some of the deterioration associated with aging. Somebody wisely said that exercise is the department with the best return on investment.

Physical activity doesn't have to be very hard, painful or extreme. You don't need to join a gym or a health club to safeguard your health.

You can improve your fitness by doing light activity for 10-minute periods. Short bouts of exercise during the course of a day have an additive benefit. That is, three 10-minute periods of exertion can be almost as beneficial as one 30-minute session. Work up to 30 minutes most, and preferably all, days of the week.

Active exercise three times a week for as little as 20 minutes a session improves your energy level, and adds to your flexibility and sense of well-being. Beginners should focus on regularity rather than intensity.

The usual question about exercise is, what kind of exercise? Scientists have recently acknowledged the value of light-to-moderate physical activity. But, what kind of activity is considered to be of moderate intensity?

All you have to do are the normal things, like walking, swimming, stair climbing, riding a bicycle, gardening, stretching, but just more often, a little longer, and a little faster.

Here is the secret to success:

When you select an exercise activity, it is important to choose something that you enjoy doing. Otherwise, you will not make it a part of your lifestyle. Devote at least 20 minutes three times a week to a physical activity that you enjoy. The secret of success lies in picking the form of exercise or a combination of them, that you would enjoy.

Is running too strenuous or boring for you?

Try WALKING:

It is the least strenuous and safest aerobic exercise and can be safely followed all the years of your life. Remember, however, for the walking to be aerobic it must be brisk. Sometimes called speed walking or power walking, this is one of the more convenient ways to exercise. All you need is a comfortable pair of walking shoes and a path.

In one test, men 40 to 57 years old walked at a fast pace for 40 minutes, four days a week and showed improvement equal to that of men of the same age who jogged for 30 minutes three days a week.

Suggestion: Start at a pace that's comfortable for you. A walk begins with slowly walking for 5 minutes to warm up then gradually pick up speed until you're walking briskly for next 5 minutes and ending with 5 minutes of walking slowly to cool down. Total time for the walk is 15 minutes. Do this every day for a week. Add five minutes to your walks next week and keep adding 5 minutes until you are walking as long as desired.

Ideas: Walk to work instead of taking public transportation or car. Take 10-15 minute brisk walk during your breaks, or before or after meals. Or simply avoid elevators—just walk up and down stairs.

Result: Within about two weeks you will notice general improvements. Your blood pressure will decrease, leg muscles will be stronger and energy levels will improve.

Walkers who wish to lose weight should gradually work up to a minimum of 5 days a week, 45 to 60 minutes or more at a moderate to vigorous intensity level (50-85% of your maximum heart rate).

Your aim: try to reach a speed of about three to five miles an hour. Walking takes more time, but it gets the same results and is safer for many people.

At first you may need to alternate walking with jogging.

Jogging:

This has been described as the most efficient way to achieve cardiovascular fitness. Jogging makes heart work less while doing more. With exercise the heart muscle's fibers lengthen and strengthen, its chambers enlarge and as a result can pump more blood with each contraction. Before training, one stroke of the heart may pump less than half a cup;

but after training, each beat may pump almost a whole cup. Because it pumps more with each beat, it beats slower and has more rest between contractions. From this training, over a period of time the heartbeats measured when you are at rest can show a decrease from 10 to 20 beats per minute. The small arteries that carry blood to the heart enlarge with training and are able to supply more oxygen-rich blood for the heart. Training also results in a gradual lowering of blood pressure.

Three days a week is preferred by many joggers for their regular training.

Do stretching exercises before and after running. Start slowly, increase gradually, don't strain.

Run in an easy and relaxed style, comfortable for you. Your pace should not leave you breathless, but able to talk as you jog.

You have no place to jog, and it's too time-consuming?

ROPE-SKIPPING:

Nothing surpasses the simple jump rope – it is the greatest fitness in the least amount of time. It can be done indoors or out. Weather is no factor. It takes less time and gives comparable results. All you'll need a four-by-six-foot area, and about 10 inches of space above your head. It is estimated that 10 minutes of jumping rope has the same benefit as jogging for 30 minutes.

To really maximize calorie burn alternate 20 seconds of work with 10 seconds of rest for four minutes. Eventually, you will move past 20 seconds, and begin working with 1, 2, and 3-minute rounds.

Try this: 5 minutes: double-leg jumps, followed by 45 seconds: plank. Then 2 minutes: single-leg jumps, 2 minutes: double-leg jumps and 45 seconds: opposite arm/leg extensions

Result: Jumping rope burns a lot of calories in a short amount of time—more than 10 calories a minute. Which means you can burn more than 200 calories in two, 10-minute sessions each day. It doesn't take long to reap major rewards—1,000 calories a week! Besides this, you will strengthen your legs, arms and shoulders. Finally, Jump rope training will enhance your coordination, agility, quickness, footwork, and endurance. It is a good stress reliever, and has the advantage of being inexpensive. For only $5, you can buy a rope that will enhance numerous physical qualities.

BICYCLING:

Medical evidence indicates that bicycling is safer than jogging for those not fit, and people have also found that it is a useful—and inexpensive means of transportation. Bicycling offers an excellent way of offsetting the harmful effects of a sedentary life.

Keep a steady pace that will make your heart work at the necessary rate to make your training aerobic.

Try this: Commit to at least 150 minutes of bicycle exercise each week. Split your exercise over at least 3 days each week. Don't just ride your bike, train!

Result: Cycling at 70 to 80% of your maximum heart rate for 15 minutes or longer helps you burn calories—up 500-700 calories an hour. Just 20 miles a week reduces your risk of heart disease to less than half that of those who take no exercise.

SWIMMING:

Practically every muscle of the body is involved in the coordinated movements of a swimmer. Fine muscle tone can be developed. Circulation is often improved, and so is the function of kidneys, bowels and other internal organs. It also helps keep your joints flexible, and it can give you virtually all the cardiovascular benefits of jogging.

All it needs is you … and a pool. Most pools are 25 yards long. Start by swimming 25 yards, then rest for 15 to 30 seconds. Repeat this pattern for 15 minutes. Then increase the distance to 50 or 75 yards. Once you feel comfortable completing these workouts, try swimming for 20 to 30 minutes. Each week you add 50 to 200 yards to your workout. You slowly build up your endurance.

Your goal: with swimming the first benchmark is a swimmer's mile, which is 1,650 yards (1,500 meters).

Result: Swimming also can be of help in improving the figure. The up and down kicking action serves to firm hips and thighs, and in time it can be a factor in trimming the waistline. The overarm movements strengthen the shoulder and back muscles, and help posture.

Word of caution: Never swim right after a meal. It could result in painful stomach cramps, which have caused even excellent swimmers to drown. Do not swim alone.

There are still other possibilities. Whatever form of exercise you choose, it must keep you moving. Its demand on the heart and lungs must be heavy, sustained and over a minimum period of time.

If a person is about 60 years of age or older physician suggest no food for 3 hours before vigorous activities and no drinking for at least 1 hour beforehand. They offer this advice: a 10-minute warm up; a 15-minute break every half-hour for fast-paced activities such as tennis; and a tepid shower afterward.

Remember: regularity is a must. It is the regularity, not just the amount, of exercise that matters. The key is not so much what you do for exercise but how often you do it. There seems to be universal agreement among scientists—if you want better health, you must exercise regularly! With that in mind, you may want to look at your calendar and schedule specific dates and times for exercise. After a few weeks of an exercise program, you will likely find that it has become a normal part of your life.

In this age of modern conveniences and machinery, many no longer have to exert themselves physically in their daily routine. Many jobs are of a sedentary nature. One only has to look at the multitudes of joggers, bicycle riders and sports enthusiasts to agree that ours has become an age in which people are trying to be aware of physical fitness.

The U.S. National Institutes of Health suggests that, "children and adults alike should set a goal of accumulating at least 30 minutes of moderate-intensity physical activity on most, and preferably all, days of the week." Like a car your health will break down if you don't maintain it properly. This involves self-discipline and good personal organization. There is no hassle-free exercise program. However, the inconveniences and sacrifices involved in maintaining an active life style pale into insignificance when compared with the life-threatening dangers of an inactive life style.

Stay active, break a sweat now and again, work those muscles—you might live a healthier and longer life! Once you begin to enjoy the health benefits, you may actually look forward to your sessions of physical activity. Yes, if exercise were a pill, it would be the most widely prescribed medication in the world.

SUPER FUEL FOODS

Burn Calories While Sleeping

Most of us, when we think of burning calories, automatically think of vigorous exercise, or an equivalent activity such as strenuous work or play, that helps us to get rid of excess fat. We do not think of the body as doing anything while we sleep. In fact, everything that we do burns calories, and that includes sleeping. One of the biggest benefits of regular exercise, in fact, is that it enhances the ability of the body to burn calories no matter what we are doing. In this article we shall explore various ways in which we can get rid of calories during the night.

The importance of sleep:

Although scientists do not yet have the answers to all questions about why we need it, the value that sleep has for our overall health—both physical and mental—cannot be overestimated. It restores energy to the body, particularly the brain and the nervous system, so that we can perform our normal activities more efficiently the next day. Scientists estimate that people spend about a third of their lives in sleep. The average adult human being should get seven or eight hours of sleep each night, though some can get by with less than six and others need more than nine. Dream sleep may be especially important if we are to learn reason, adjust emotionally and perform other mental activities more efficiently.

The amount of sleep that we get profoundly affects the way we eat and our desire to exercise, both of which in turn influence the body's capacity for burning fat. When we sleep properly, two hormones that regulate hunger—ghrelin and lepton—are released at their proper times and in their proper proportions. Ghrelin is what makes us feel hungry when we have not eaten, while lepton makes us feel full when that need has been satisfied. Too little sleep causes the balance of these hormones to be disrupted. Excessive amounts of ghrelin and too little lepton are released so that the body always feels hungry and the person ends up overeating.

How sleep burns calories:

Several bodily activities that occur during sleep burn fat. The muscles burn more calories when they are at rest, and this is especially true for those who have a high amount of muscle mass and therefore burn more sugar and fat. Fit Day says that one pound of muscle uses up 50 calories for a single day. A pound of fat, on the other hand, consumes no more than 9 calories. For that reason, you should work out regularly with weights to develop muscle tissue, while at the same time engaging in aerobic exercise to burn fat. Both these things will increase your basal metabolic rate, the amount of energy that an organism expends during rest.

It is a good idea to exercise early in the day in order to "jump start" the system for the remainder of your waking hours. Likewise you should cease all workout activity at least a few hours before you get into bed. Depending on the weather or the season, you might also want to have breakfast outside in the sun, which can reset your "biological clock." If you find yourself feeling drowsy during the day, consider taking a nap for 10 or 20 minutes.

Foods that help you burn calories while sleeping:

Our ability to burn calories while we sleep depends on the foods that we eat. Total Health Guide, a

British online magazine, has recommended five foods that are especially good for that purpose.

Almonds

Almonds contain what are often incorrectly thought to be "negative calories," meaning that they require more energy to digest than they provide. There is no scientific evidence to prove that such is the case, but almonds do indeed increase the diligence of the body during sleep, particularly if you eat a handful of them just before you go to bed. Other nuts include pistachios, Brazil nuts, walnuts, hazel nuts and pine nuts.

Bananas

The banana, which is high in potassium and fiber, is one of the most nourishing foods that you can eat. If you have one as a bedtime snack—and you should eat it by itself, with no biscuits or anything else whatsoever—it will put your metabolism to work through the night and make you wake up in the morning with a sense of hunger.

Blueberries

Blueberries are another food that is said to have "negative calories." Other such fruits include blackberries, cherries, nectarines, plums, raspberries

118

and strawberries. They will all help you to get a good night's sleep.

Carrots

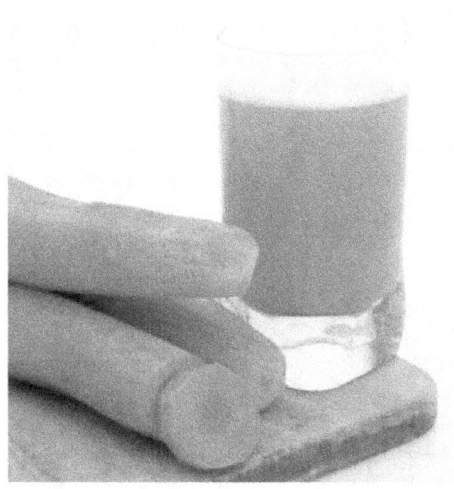

The carrot is especially good for the teeth, but it is also an excellent nighttime snack. The carotene that it contains converts into vitamin A, which then sets of a chain reaction that rids the body of its excess fat. Best of all, it has only 30 calories.

Yogurt

Yogurt is a milk product that was first made in Turkey and other parts of the Middle East thousands of years ago (indeed, yogurt is a Turkish word; for those who are interested it comes from an obsolete word meaning to curdle or thicken.) Many people who on a low-calorie diet like to eat unflavored yogurt, which has only a few calories in each serving. Better still, yogurt contains probiotic ingredients that improve the functioning of the digestive tract. If taken at night it will force the body to burn more calories than it otherwise would. It is also an excellent source of animal protein and calcium, which play a large part in muscular growth.

One of the benefits of having a pre-bedtime snack is that it keeps the body from entering into a catatonic state, in which the starving system obtains the fuel it needs by feeding into the muscles.

How to calculate the number of calories you burn in your sleep:

Normally the body burns 0.42 calories per hour per pound. If you weigh 143 pounds, for instance, you should burn 60.06 calories per hour, which amounts to 48.58 during an eight-hour night of sleep. Finally, the more calories you burn at night, the more you burn during the day.

QUESTIONS AND ANSWERS

There are many fads, myths, half-truths and elaborate lies that surround weight loss and unfortunately many people believe and implement these falsehoods into their regimens and as a result do not achieve the progress promised. My job is to answer some of the most common questions surrounding weight loss that people are too afraid or ashamed to ask because they believe the questions are stupid or the answers are obvious. When it comes to our bodies the words 'stupid' and 'obvious' should not be uttered, and hopefully these answers will alleviate any doubts you have and guide you on losing those pesky pounds.

How often should I weigh myself?

Weighing yourself is important to determine how well your diet is progressing. It is recommended that you weigh yourself once a week, preferably in the morning before you have eaten. If you are more comfortable weighing yourself more frequently, for instance twice a week or less frequent like once a month, then that is fine as well.

Can I eat sweets even though I am dieting?

I think it is safe to say that we are all kids in a candy store and getting yourself to quit eating candy once you begin dieting is irrational. Candy is fine as long as it is eaten in moderation. Check the candy bar and ensure that it is less than 150 calories; trust me, there are plenty of healthy sweet options out there.

Can I lose calories by skipping meals?

This question is often asked by brides who want to lose a pound or 2 before the big day. To them I say yes, skipping meals will shed a few pounds in the short term but if you continue skipping meals you will face serious physical and emotional deficits and the only way to reverse this is to eat more than usual. I would not recommend this as a weight loss regimen.

How long does it take to lose weight?

The rate of weight loss differs among different people. Age, original weight, diet and workout regimen are all factors. Losing 1 to 2 pounds a week is an achievable and healthy option and should be used to determine how long it will take you to reach your desired weight. Remember, rapid weight loss is not advisable as your joints and muscles may experience some damage.

Which low calorie foods are the most filling?

Many people are scared that going on a diet means feeling hungry most of the time, I am happy to say that this is a myth. The following foods contain low calories but are filling: fruits, beans, vegetables, fish, turkey, chicken, whole grains, soups and low-fat dairy.

How do I maintain my desired weight?

The journey is not over when you get to your desired weight; you have to work to keep your weight. You can maintain your weight by surrounding yourself with the same foods you ate during your diet and exercising for at least an hour a day.

What foods and drinks should I stay away from as I try and lose weight?

You should avoid the following:; alcohol, as it slows down your metabolism, salt leads to water retention and thus water weight, artificial sugars and carbonated drinks have sugar which is usually converted to fat in your body. Fatty and processed foods should be completely cut out of your diet.

How many calories should I consume a day when trying to lose weight?

It is difficult to place a definite amount on the calories one should consume per day as age, gender, height, size; health and lifestyle need to be put into play. However, 2,500 calories for men and 2,000 calories for women can be used as a baseline. Thirty-five hundred calories are equal to one pound, and if your goal is to lose a pound week, eliminate 3,500 calories from your diet.

Is eating 100 calories of candy equal to eating 100 calories of fruit?

Yes; however, the sugar in fruit is good and will burn off fast while the sugar in candy is more likely to be converted into fat. Fruit is the more nutritious option.

How many meals should I eat a day?

It is recommended that one should eat five to six small meals a day as this helps the body become more efficient in burning food and prevents long stretches of hunger that usually result in overeating.

What fun activities can you do to lose weight?

I do admit that many of the exercise machines we see at the gym look scary, daunting and most importantly boring. Keeping this in mind exercise does not have to be boring; it can be tailored to your likes ensuring that you enjoy shedding off those pounds. Dancing, hiking, walking the dog, pillow fights and rock climbing are some of the ways to switch up your routine.

Why am I exercising but still gaining weight?

The obvious answers are lack of sleep, stress, medications and inefficient exercise regimens; however, a few other factors can explain your weight gain. Efficient workouts can lead to increases in water weight and muscle mass and therefore weight gain. Gaining weight is not always a bad thing.

Why is drinking water important when losing weight?

Dehydration slows down your metabolism and drinking water prevents this. Additionally, drinking water flushes out the toxins the body gains when burning calories as well as eliminates any possibility of constipation; poop adds weight to your body. Lastly, water reduces muscle and joint soreness, making it easier for you to exercise.

Why is breakfast important?

Breakfast is the most important meal of the day for a good reason; it gives you energy which makes you more active throughout the day, provides you with a brain boost and most importantly it makes you happy—people who skip breakfast tend to be irritable and cranky, and we don't like that.

Can I have a 'cheat day'?

As tempting as it is to recommend cheat days, the setbacks can be monumental. You may eat 1,000-2,000 calories more than usual. I discourage cheat days, but I believe you can incorporate some of your cravings into your diet without posing a risk to your weight loss regimen. Have a low-calorie candy bar, nibble on low-fat chips and eat a slice of pizza with low-fat cheese.

I hope all of your queries have been answered to your satisfaction. All that is left is for you to grab a friend and have massive amounts of fun shedding those pesky pounds.

A brief note:

If the contents I presented in this book were useful to you in any way, the best compliment you can provide me is a good review. This will allow my books to get into more people's hands and, together, we can help other reach our goals. Thank you,

Pennie Mae Cartawick

About the author

Pennie Mae Cartawick was born in the city of Sheffield in South Yorkshire, England. Shortly after graduating high school, she worked as a model and attended Shirecliffe College for Drama. Thereafter, she attended Stannington College for English, Art, Communication Skills and Photography. She then moved to London in her early twenties, where she studied and attained a career as a Beauty Therapist. She also obtained various certifications at DaneGlow International for slimming wraps and other deep heat treatments, and Thalgo Cosmetics for makeup (a French Company focusing on marine cosmetics). Her specialized skills include makeup, Swedish massage, reflexology, nutrition, diet and exercise.

She migrated to Florida in 1993, where she has been living ever since. Although her profession now-a-days is as a real estate investor and a freelance beauty consultant, her passion is writing, and she uses the knowledge she acquired throughout the years on various subjects to enlighten others.

She is the youngest sibling of three, including Anthony and Mark Cartawick.